KIDNEY STONE DIET FOR SENIORS

An Experts Comprehensive insight on Preventing and Treating Incurable Kidney stones completely.

Richie Smile Walker

Disclaimer

This publication is designed to provide competent and reliable information regarding the subject covered. However, the views expressed in this publication are those of the author alone, and should not be taken as expert instruction or professional advice. The reader is responsible for his or her actions. The author hereby disclaims any responsibility or liability whatsoever that is incurred from the use or application of the contents of this publication by the purchaser of the reader. The purchaser or reader is hereby responsible for his or her actions.

Copyright © 2024

Table of Contents

Introduction

Embarking upon the senior years signifies the commencement of a chapter characterized by wisdom, accumulated experiences, and contemplative reflection. Within the tapestry of these golden years, the looming presence of kidney stones can cast a shadow over the pursuit of overall well-being. It is against this backdrop that "Kidney Stone Diet for Seniors" emerges, not merely as a guide but as a meticulously crafted companion. This companion is dedicated to empowering and enlightening seniors about the intricate relationship between their dietary choices and the prevention of kidney stones.

Understanding Kidney Stones

The journey unfolds with a fundamental exploration into the realm of kidney stones, a crystalline phenomenon that demands attention. This section meticulously unravels the various types and characteristics of kidney stones, offering seniors invaluable insights. By delving into the intricacies of calcium oxalate, uric acid, struvite, and cystine stones, seniors are equipped with a nuanced understanding. The guide becomes a beacon, shedding light on the landscape of risk factors and symptoms. Seniors embark on this informational odyssey, laying the bedrock for informed decision-making in their unique health journey.

The Role of Diet in Kidney Stone Prevention for Seniors

Crucially, the guide pivots to the central theme—the pivotal role of diet in preventing kidney stones for seniors. This section acts as a tailored lens, guiding seniors through considerations such as calcium intake, the significance of hydration, and the subtle influence of sodium in their dietary choices. Recognizing that the dietary landscape evolves with age, the guide becomes a compass, aiding seniors in navigating this evolving terrain.

In the subsequent chapters, the guide delves into the intricate realm of key nutrients essential for kidney health. It unfolds a tapestry of dietary guidelines, intricately woven to resonate with the unique needs and considerations of seniors. The exploration extends to practical meal planning strategies, offering more than mere information—it provides a roadmap towards sustained well-being.

"Kidney Stone Diet for Seniors" transcends its role as a guide; it metamorphoses into a companion on the journey towards optimal health. It becomes an ally, ensuring that seniors not only understand but also embrace a lifestyle where they can savor their golden years unencumbered by the specter of kidney stones. It stands as a testament to the commitment to enhancing the quality of life for seniors, making their well-being a priority, and providing them with the tools to navigate this chapter with vitality and resilience.

CHAPTER 1:

TYPES OF KIDNEY STONES

In the vast landscape of kidney health, it's essential for seniors on their journey toward well-being to grasp the intricacies of various kidney stones. Each type comes with its unique characteristics, causes, and considerations. This chapter serves as a guide, shedding light on the four primary types: Calcium Oxalate Stones, Uric Acid Stones, Struvite Stones, and Cystine Stones.

Calcium Oxalate Stones

Formation and Characteristics

Let's start with the most common kidney stone—calcium oxalate stones. They form when there's an imbalance in calcium and oxalate levels in urine. Oxalate, found in many foods, combines with calcium, creating crystals that can aggregate into these stones. Visualizing them, they often look like hard, crystalline structures of varying sizes. Several factors, including dietary habits, genetics, and hydration levels, influence their formation.

Risk Factors and Prevention Strategies

Seniors need to be aware of risk factors like a diet high in oxalate-rich foods, inadequate fluid intake, and specific medical conditions. To prevent calcium oxalate stones, dietary adjustments are crucial—

reducing the intake of oxalate-rich foods such as spinach, nuts, and beets. Hydration plays a pivotal role, diluting the concentration of oxalate and calcium in urine.

Uric Acid Stones

Formation and Characteristics

Moving on to uric acid stones, these develop when there's an excess of uric acid in urine, forming crystals. Seniors may be prone to these due to dietary choices, age-related metabolic changes, or conditions like gout. Uric acid stones often have a smooth, yellow-brown appearance and can vary in size.

Risk Factors and Prevention Strategies

Understanding the formation process is crucial for seniors managing or preventing uric acid stones. Factors like a diet rich in purines found in certain meats and seafood, along with age-related metabolic changes, contribute to their increased risk. Prevention involves dietary modifications, including reducing purine-rich foods and ensuring proper hydration to prevent uric acid concentration in urine.

Struvite Stones

Formation and Characteristics

Struvite stones, also known as infection stones, form in the presence of urinary tract infections caused by specific bacteria. Composed of magnesium, ammonium, and phosphate, these stones may affect seniors with a history of recurrent urinary tract infections, a common concern in older individuals. Struvite stones are known for their rapid growth and tendency to form large, branched structures.

Risk Factors and Prevention Strategies

Seniors need to be vigilant about urinary tract infections as they can lead to struvite stone formation. Prevention strategies revolve around promptly treating urinary tract infections to inhibit stone formation. Maintaining good hygiene practices and seeking medical attention for signs of infection are crucial in preventing struvite stones among seniors.

Cystine Stones

Formation and Characteristics

Cystine stones, a rare type, result from the accumulation of the amino acid cystine in urine, often due to a hereditary condition called cystinuria. Seniors with a family history of cystinuria face an increased risk. These stones are characterized by their hexagonal shape and relatively smooth surface and tend to be larger and more resistant to common preventive measures.

Risk Factors and Prevention Strategies

Seniors with a familial history of cystinuria should be aware of the increased risk of cystine stones. Prevention involves a combination of dietary modifications and medications to reduce cystine levels in urine. Adequate hydration is crucial to prevent the concentration of cystine in the urinary tract.

Understanding the various types of kidney stones is essential for seniors looking to proactively manage kidney health. Each stone type requires a personalized approach to prevention, emphasizing dietary choices, hydration, and awareness of individual risk factors. This chapter serves as a compass, guiding seniors through the intricacies of kidney stone prevention with practical insights and a commitment to their well-being.

CHAPTER 2

DIAGNOSTIC OVERVIEW

For seniors, navigating the world of kidney stones is vital for their well-being. In Chapter 2 of "Kidney Stone Diet for Seniors," we explore a straightforward overview of diagnosis, covering identifying risk factors, recognizing symptoms, and the crucial role of dietary management in prevention.

Spotting Kidney Stone Risk Factors

Family Connections

When it comes to identifying kidney stone risks, understanding family history is key. If there's a history of specific stones like cystine stones, seniors can take proactive steps to mitigate risks.

The Aging Equation

Seniors naturally face a higher risk due to changes in metabolism and kidney function as they age. Recognizing these age-related factors lays the groundwork for targeted preventive approaches, emphasizing the need to adjust dietary habits to align with the changing needs of aging bodies.

Health Conditions and Medications

Certain health conditions, such as chronic kidney disease, and medications like diuretics, can elevate the risk of kidney stones. Recognizing these factors empowers seniors to have informed discussions with healthcare professionals, ensuring a holistic approach to overall health.

Understanding Symptoms and Diagnosis

Recognizing Signs

In the journey to prevent kidney stones, being aware of common symptoms is crucial. Seniors should be attentive to signs like severe back or abdominal pain, blood in urine, and changes in urinary frequency. Early recognition of these symptoms plays a vital role in timely diagnosis and intervention.

Diagnostic Tools

The diagnostic process involves various tools, including imaging techniques like CT scans and ultrasounds, providing a visual representation of kidney stones. Urinalysis offers insights into urine composition and potential risk factors. These tools collectively contribute to a thorough diagnosis, guiding healthcare professionals in developing appropriate preventive strategies.

The Value of Regular Check-ups

Regular medical check-ups become a cornerstone in the diagnostic process for seniors. These check-ups enable healthcare professionals to monitor kidney function, assess risk factors, and identify emerging symptoms. Seniors are encouraged to actively engage in their healthcare journey, fostering open communication with healthcare providers for a proactive and personalized approach to diagnosis.

Dietary Management: A Personalized Approach

Tailoring Diets to Stone Types

Dietary management takes center stage in preventing kidney stones among seniors. Understanding the specific types of kidney stones allows for personalized dietary choices. For example, those prone to calcium oxalate stones may benefit from moderating oxalate-rich foods, while individuals at risk of uric acid stones should consider reducing purines in their diet.

The Role of Hydration

Adequate hydration is a cornerstone in kidney stone prevention. Seniors are advised to maintain a consistent and sufficient fluid intake to dilute the concentration of minerals in urine, reducing the likelihood of stone formation. Hydration becomes a simple yet powerful tool in the dietary toolkit against kidney stones.

Finding Moderation and Balance

Dietary management emphasizes moderation and balance, promoting a varied and nutrient-rich diet while considering individual risk factors. Seniors are encouraged to collaborate with healthcare professionals or dieticians to create personalized meal plans aligned with their preferences and health needs.

Monitoring and Adaptation

Continual monitoring of dietary habits and their impact on kidney health is vital for preventive care. Seniors are urged to keep a close eye on their diets, making adjustments as needed based on diagnostic findings and evolving health conditions. This adaptive approach ensures that dietary management remains a dynamic and responsive aspect of kidney stone prevention.

CHAPTER 3

EATING RIGHT TO KEEP KIDNEY STONES AWAY

In Chapter 3 of "Kidney Stone Diet for Seniors," we're breaking down the essentials of eating smart to safeguard those precious kidneys. This chapter is all about what seniors need to know when it comes to nutrition for preventing kidney stones. We'll cover the must-have nutrients, the magic of staying hydrated, and the role sodium plays in the formation of those pesky stones.

Nutrients that Keep Kidneys Happy

Calcium: Friend, Not Foe

Let's clear the air about calcium—it's not the bad guy. It's a key player in preventing kidney stones. Seniors, we'll explore the sweet spot for calcium intake because too much or too little can tip the scales toward stone formation. Say goodbye to myths and hello to the real scoop on optimizing calcium for kidney health.

Magnesium: The Silent Supporter

Meet magnesium, the unsung hero often overshadowed by calcium. Seniors, let's dive into how magnesium steps up to prevent calcium oxalate stones. It's all about understanding the dance between these minerals for top-notch kidney health.

Vitamin D: Soaking in the Sun

Vitamin D isn't just for bones—it's a VIP for kidney health too. Seniors, we'll explore where to get this sunshine vitamin, how it teams up with calcium, and the delicate balance needed to reap the benefits without causing trouble with kidney stones.

Hydration: Your Kidneys' Best Friend

Hydration Power Play

Here's the golden ticket to preventing kidney stones—hydration. Seniors, we'll dig into how keeping those fluids flowing reduces the risk of stone formation. Forget the routine; think of hydration as your kidney's lifeline, and we'll guide you through practical strategies tailored to the unique challenges you might face.

Sipping Smart: Hydration Hacks

Seniors, aging can throw some curveballs at hydration levels. No worries—we've got your back with tailored strategies. From sipping water throughout the day to munching on hydrating foods, we'll spill the beans on keeping your fluid balance in check.

Beyond Water: Beverage Breakdown

Let's talk beverages—some are hydrating heroes, while others might be villains. Seniors, we'll spill the tea on herbal goodness and flag the sugary foes. Armed with this knowledge, you'll make choices that not only keep you hydrated but also kick those kidney stones to the curb.

Sodium: The Sneaky Stone Culprit

Sodium Unmasked: The Culprit Revealed

Sodium, the sneaky character hiding in processed foods, has a role in kidney stone formation. Seniors, we'll unveil the mechanisms through which high sodium levels can up the stone risk, especially if you're prone to calcium-containing stones. This section demystifies sodium, giving you the power to make dietary choices that keep taste intact without compromising nutrition.

Smart Sodium Moves: Reducing the Salt Without Losing Flavor

Seniors, practical tips for cutting back on sodium without sacrificing taste take center stage here. From deciphering labels to jazz up your meals with herbs and spices, we'll equip you with actionable steps for a kidney-friendly approach to sodium.

Balance Act: Sodium and Fluid Harmony

Ever wondered how sodium plays with fluid balance? Seniors, we're diving into the intricate relationship between sodium and your body's water retention. Understanding this delicate balance ensures that your sodium intake aligns to prevent kidney stones.

List of foods that seniors can include in their diet

Ensuring a diet that promotes kidney health is vital, especially for seniors aiming to prevent kidney stones. Below is a detailed list of foods that seniors can include in their diet to support their kidneys and minimize the risk of kidney stones:

1. Water:

Explanation: Keeping well-hydrated is crucial to prevent kidney stones. Water aids in diluting minerals and substances in urine, reducing the likelihood of stone formation.

2. Citrus Fruits:

Examples: Oranges, lemons, limes, grapefruits.

Explanation: Citrus fruits are loaded with citrate, which helps thwart the development of specific types of kidney stones by binding to calcium in urine.

3. Berries:

Examples: Strawberries, blueberries, raspberries.

Explanation: Berries are both low in oxalates and high in antioxidants, making them an excellent choice for kidney stone prevention.

4. Apples:

Explanation: Apples are low in oxalates and high in dietary fiber, promoting overall digestive health.

5. Watermelon:

Explanation: Watermelon, with its high water content, aids in hydration and contains citrulline, potentially preventing kidney stone formation.

6. Cucumbers:

Explanation: Cucumbers are hydrating and low in oxalates, providing a refreshing and kidney-friendly snack.

7. Bell Peppers:

Explanation: Low in oxalates and rich in vitamins A and C, bell peppers are a nutritious addition to the diet.

8. Cauliflower:

Explanation: Cauliflower, being a low-oxalate cruciferous vegetable, offers essential nutrients without contributing to stone formation.

9. Grapes:

Explanation: Grapes, especially red and purple varieties, contain compounds that may lower the risk of kidney stones.

10. Pineapple:

Explanation: Pineapple is not only flavorful but also contains bromelain, an enzyme with potential anti-inflammatory properties.

11. Red Bell Peppers:

Explanation: Low in oxalates and high in vitamins A and C, red bell peppers support overall health.

12. Olive Oil:

Explanation: Olive oil, a healthy fat for cooking or dressing salads, provides monounsaturated fats and antioxidants.

13. Fish:

Examples: Salmon, trout.

Explanation: Fatty fish rich in omega-3 fatty acids may have anti-inflammatory effects, promoting heart and kidney health.

14. Low-Fat Dairy:

Examples: Low-fat yogurt, skim milk.

Explanation: Low-fat dairy is a good calcium source without increasing the risk of kidney stones.

15. Eggs:

Explanation: Eggs are a high-quality protein source suitable for a kidney stone prevention diet.

16. Whole Grains:

Examples: Brown rice, quinoa, whole wheat.

Explanation: Whole grains offer fiber and nutrients without contributing to oxalate levels.

17. Lean Proteins:

Examples: Chicken, turkey, lean beef.

Explanation: Lean protein sources are crucial for a balanced diet without elevating the risk of kidney stones.

18. Herbs and Spices:

Examples: Basil, thyme, ginger.

Explanation: Herbs and spices enhance flavor without adding oxalates to dishes.

19. Dark Chocolate (in moderation):

Explanation: Dark chocolate, in moderation, provides antioxidants without significantly increasing the risk of kidney stones.

20. Herbal Teas:

Examples: Chamomile, peppermint.

Explanation: Herbal teas offer hydration and varied flavors without introducing oxalates.

List of foods that seniors can limit in their diet

Avoiding certain foods is crucial for seniors with kidney stones. Here's a clear and understandable list along with explanations:

1. High-Oxalate Foods:

Examples: Spinach, beets, nuts, chocolate.

Explanation: These foods are rich in oxalates, which can lead to the formation of calcium oxalate stones. Reducing intake helps manage oxalate levels.

2. Processed Foods:

Examples: Canned soups, instant noodles, packaged snacks.

Explanation: Processed foods often have high sodium and additives, increasing the risk of kidney stone formation. Opt for whole, natural foods.

3. Red Meat:

Examples: Beef, lamb, pork.

Explanation: Red meat contains purines, contributing to the formation of uric acid stones. Moderation is essential to manage this risk.

4. Organ Meats:

Examples: Liver, kidney, heart.

Explanation: Organ meats have high purine content, elevating uric acid levels and increasing the risk of uric acid stones. Limit consumption.

5. Sugary Beverages:

Examples: Soda, energy drinks, sweetened juices.

Explanation: High sugar intake can lead to dehydration and increase the risk of stone formation. Opt for water or herbal teas.

6. Excessive Caffeine:

Examples: Coffee, tea, and energy drinks.

Explanation: Caffeine can contribute to dehydration, potentially leading to concentrated urine and stone formation. Consume caffeine in moderation.

7. High-Sodium Foods:

Examples: Processed meats, canned soups, fast food.

Explanation: High sodium levels increase calcium excretion in urine, contributing to stone formation. Choose low-sodium alternatives.

8. Colas and Carbonated Drinks:

Explanation: Colas contain phosphoric acid, which may increase the risk of kidney stones. Additionally, the caffeine content can contribute to dehydration.

9. Excessive Dairy:

Examples: Full-fat dairy products.

Explanation: While moderate calcium intake is essential, excessive consumption of full-fat dairy may increase the risk of calcium oxalate stones.

10. Certain Vegetables:

Examples: Beets, okra, sweet potatoes.

Explanation: Vegetables high in oxalates should be consumed in moderation to manage oxalate levels.

11. High-Protein Diets:

Explanation: Diets excessively high in protein, especially animal proteins, may increase the risk of kidney stones. Balance protein intake with other nutrients.

12. Excessive Vitamin C Supplements:

Explanation: High doses of vitamin C supplements may be converted into oxalates in the body, potentially increasing the risk of stone formation.

13. Alcohol:

Explanation: Alcohol can lead to dehydration, concentrating urine, and promoting stone formation. Moderation is advised.

14. Certain Fish:

Examples: Sardines, anchovies.

Explanation: These fish are high in purines, contributing to the risk of uric acid stone formation. Limit their consumption.

CHAPTER 4

DIETARY GUIDELINES FOR KIDNEY STONE PREVENTION

"Kidney Stone Diet for Seniors" becomes your trustworthy guide. Forget the jargon; we're here to lead seniors through the maze of dietary choices that can make all the difference. This section covers the real deal about a low oxalate diet, smart strategies for getting enough calcium, understanding the link between purine-rich foods and uric acid stones, and finding the right balance between acidic and alkaline foods.

Low Oxalate Diet: Sorting Myth from Reality

Decoding Oxalates

Let's cut through the confusion around oxalates. Seniors, it's not about banishing them entirely; it's about making informed choices. We'll break down the facts, identify foods high in oxalates, and arm you with practical tips for a balanced approach that doesn't require extremes.

Oxalates and Calcium Dance

Understanding how oxalates and calcium tango in your body is crucial. Seniors, we'll dive into the interaction and why finding the right balance matters. This part unveils insights into optimizing calcium intake without falling into the trap of too little calcium, which can actually up the risk of certain kidney stones.

Calcium Intake Strategies: Getting the Goldilocks Amount

Calcium's Double Duty

Seniors, calcium is more than just a bone supporter—it plays a big role in warding off certain kidney stones. This section unveils the dual nature of calcium and spills the beans on how smart intake can be a game-changer. No more calcium confusion; we're providing practical strategies to ensure you hit the sweet spot.

Where to Find Calcium Goodies

Wondering where to get your calcium fix? Seniors, we're laying out the buffet of calcium sources, from dairy delights to plant-powered options. Whether you're saying no to lactose or cheering for dairy, we've got the lowdown on diverse sources to fit your taste.

Purine-Rich Foods and Uric Acid Stones: Navigating the Landscape

The Purine Story

Seniors, let's chat about purines—the players in the uric acid stone game. No need to worry; we're not banishing tasty treats. We'll explore the purine world, identify foods with high purine content, and understand how they connect to uric acid stones. Knowledge is your power, and we're handing you the reins for informed choices.

Finding Balance: Smart Purine Choices

Practical tips take the spotlight as we navigate the tightrope of enjoying purine-rich foods without inviting uric acid stones to the party. Seniors, from moderating your intake to bringing purine-friendly options into the mix, we're laying out a roadmap for a balanced approach that aligns with your taste buds and keeps your kidneys happy.

Acidic and Alkaline Foods Balance: A Symphony for Kidney Health

The pH Mystery

Seniors, let's unravel the mystery of pH—understanding how foods' acidity and alkalinity impact kidney health. We'll sift through myths and truths, offering insights into how balancing these elements can play a role in preventing stones. No more confusion; say hello to a harmonious dietary approach.

Acidic Foods and Stone Formation

Certain foods can tilt the pH scale towards acidity, potentially affecting stone formation. Seniors, we'll shed light on these culprits and discuss moderation strategies. It's not about saying goodbye to them but making informed choices that maintain the delicate balance.

Discover the alkaline side of the food spectrum. Seniors, we're highlighting foods that lean towards the alkaline side, potentially lending support to kidney health. From fruits to veggies, we're offering a list of alkaline allies and practical tips to seamlessly weave them into your diet.

CHAPTER 5

MEAL PLANNING FOR KIDNEY STONE PREVENTION

Here's a 30-day meal plan for seniors focusing on kidney stone-friendly foods and avoiding those that may contribute to stone formation:

Day 1:

Breakfast:

- Scrambled eggs with spinach (limited) and whole-grain toast.
- Citrus fruit salad (oranges and berries).

Lunch:

- Grilled chicken salad with mixed greens, bell peppers, and olive oil dressing.
- Watermelon slices.

Dinner:

- Baked salmon with lemon and herbs.
- Steamed cauliflower.
- Quinoa.

Day 2:

Breakfast:

- Greek yogurt with sliced apples.
- Herbal tea.

Lunch:

- Turkey and vegetable wrap with a whole wheat tortilla.
- Cucumber slices.

Dinner:

- Stir-fried tofu with mixed vegetables.
- Brown rice.

Day 3:

Breakfast:

- Oatmeal with berries and a sprinkle of chopped nuts (limited).
- Orange juice.

Lunch:

- Lentil soup with plenty of vegetables.
- Fresh pineapple chunks.

Dinner:

- Grilled shrimp skewers with a side of steamed broccoli.

- Quinoa.

Day 4:

Breakfast:

- Cottage cheese with sliced peaches.
- Chamomile tea.

Lunch:

- Spinach and feta-stuffed chicken breast.
- Mixed berry salad.

Dinner:

- Vegetable curry with chickpeas.
- Cauliflower rice.

Day 5:

Breakfast:

- Smoothie with berries, bananas, and almond milk.
- Whole grain toast with a thin spread of almond butter.

Lunch:

- Quinoa salad with tomatoes, cucumbers, and feta cheese.
- Orange slices.

Dinner:

- Grilled trout with lemon and dill.

- Steamed asparagus.
- Brown rice.

Day 6:

Breakfast:

- Scrambled eggs with tomatoes and herbs.
- Herbal tea.

Lunch:

- Tuna salad with mixed greens.
- Sliced cucumber.

Dinner:

- Stir-fried vegetables with tofu.
- Quinoa.

Day 7:

Breakfast:

- Overnight oats with mixed berries.
- Fresh orange juice.

Lunch:

- Chicken and vegetable stir-fry.
- Watermelon slices.

Dinner:

- Baked cod with a squeeze of lemon.
- Steamed broccoli.
- Cauliflower rice.

Day 8:

Breakfast:

- Whole grain cereal with low-fat milk.
- Sliced peaches.

Lunch:

- Turkey and avocado whole grain wrap.
- Mixed berry salad.

Dinner:

- Grilled chicken breast with a squeeze of lemon.
- Steamed green beans.
- Quinoa.

Day 9:

Breakfast:

- Smoothie with spinach, banana, and low-fat yogurt.
- Whole grain toast with a thin spread of almond butter.

Lunch:

- Lentil and vegetable soup.

- Fresh pineapple chunks.

Dinner:

- Baked tilapia with herbs.

- Roasted Brussels sprouts.

- Brown rice.

Day 10:

Breakfast:

- Scrambled eggs with tomatoes and herbs.

- Herbal tea.

Lunch:

- Chickpea salad with cherry tomatoes and feta cheese.

- Sliced cucumber.

Dinner:

- Stir-fried tofu with broccoli and bell peppers.

- Quinoa.

Day 11:

Breakfast:

- Greek yogurt with sliced strawberries.

- Orange juice.

Lunch:

- Chicken and vegetable kebabs.
- Watermelon slices.

Dinner:

- Grilled salmon with a side of asparagus.
- Cauliflower rice.

Day 12:

Breakfast:

- Oatmeal with sliced bananas and a sprinkle of chopped nuts (limited).
- Chamomile tea.

Lunch:

- Spinach and feta-stuffed portobello mushrooms.
- Fresh berries.

Dinner:

- Vegetable stir-fry with tofu.
- Brown rice.

Day 13:

Breakfast:

- Cottage cheese with mixed berries.
- Herbal tea.

Lunch:

- Quinoa and black bean salad.
- Sliced orange.

Dinner:

- Grilled shrimp with lemon and garlic.
- Steamed broccoli.
- Quinoa.

Day 14:

Breakfast:

- Banana and almond milk smoothie.
- Whole grain toast with a thin spread of cream cheese.

Lunch:

- Turkey and vegetable stir-fry.
- Mixed berry salad.

Dinner:

- Baked chicken with rosemary.

- Roasted sweet potatoes.

- Cauliflower rice.

Day 15:

Breakfast:

- Yogurt parfait with fresh berries and a sprinkle of granola.

- Herbal tea.

Lunch:

- Quinoa and vegetable stuffed bell peppers.

- Sliced cucumber.

Dinner:

- Grilled tilapia with a squeeze of lime.

- Steamed asparagus.

- Brown rice.

Day 16:

Breakfast:

- Scrambled eggs with diced tomatoes and spinach.

- Whole grain toast with a thin spread of peanut butter.

Lunch:

- Lentil soup with a side of sliced oranges.

- Mixed berry salad.

Dinner:

- Baked chicken breast with herbs.
- Roasted Brussels sprouts.
- Quinoa.

Day 17:

Breakfast:

- Smoothie with kale, banana, and low-fat yogurt.
- Whole grain toast with a thin spread of almond butter.

Lunch:

- Turkey and avocado wrap with a side of sliced melon.
- Mixed vegetable sticks.

Dinner:

- Stir-fried tofu with broccoli and snow peas.
- Brown rice.

Day 18:

Breakfast:

- Greek yogurt with sliced strawberries.
- Orange juice.

Lunch:

- Chickpea salad with cherry tomatoes and feta cheese.

* Sliced cucumber.

Dinner:

* Grilled salmon with a lemon herb marinade.
* Quinoa.

Day 19:

Breakfast:

* Oatmeal with sliced bananas and a sprinkle of chopped nuts (limited).
* Chamomile tea.

Lunch:

* Spinach and feta-stuffed portobello mushrooms.
* Fresh berries.

Dinner:

* Vegetable stir-fry with tofu.
* Cauliflower rice.

Day 20:

Breakfast:

* Cottage cheese with mixed berries.
* Herbal tea.

Lunch:

- Quinoa and black bean salad.
- Sliced orange.

Dinner:

- Grilled shrimp with lemon and garlic.
- Steamed broccoli.
- Quinoa.

Day 21:

Breakfast:

- Banana and almond milk smoothie.
- Whole grain toast with a thin spread of cream cheese.

Lunch:

- Turkey and vegetable stir-fry.
- Mixed berry salad.

Dinner:

- Baked chicken with rosemary.
- Roasted sweet potatoes.
- Cauliflower rice.

Day 22:

Breakfast:

- Scrambled eggs with diced tomatoes and spinach.
- Whole grain toast with a thin spread of almond butter.

Lunch:

- Lentil soup with a side of sliced oranges.
- Mixed berry salad.

Dinner:

- Baked chicken breast with herbs.
- Roasted Brussels sprouts.
- Quinoa.

Day 23:

Breakfast:

- Smoothie with kale, banana, and low-fat yogurt.
- Whole grain toast with a thin spread of peanut butter.

Lunch:

- Turkey and avocado wrap with a side of sliced melon.
- Mixed vegetable sticks.

Dinner:

- Stir-fried tofu with broccoli and snow peas.

- Brown rice.

Day 24:

Breakfast:

- Greek yogurt with sliced strawberries.
- Orange juice.

Lunch:

- Chickpea salad with cherry tomatoes and feta cheese.
- Sliced cucumber.

Dinner:

- Grilled salmon with a lemon herb marinade.
- Quinoa.

Day 25:

Breakfast:

- Oatmeal with sliced bananas and a sprinkle of chopped nuts (limited).
- Chamomile tea.

Lunch:

- Spinach and feta-stuffed portobello mushrooms.
- Fresh berries.

Dinner:

- Vegetable stir-fry with tofu.
- Cauliflower rice.

Day 26:

Breakfast:

- Cottage cheese with mixed berries.
- Herbal tea.

Lunch:

- Quinoa and black bean salad.
- Sliced orange.

Dinner:

- Grilled shrimp with lemon and garlic.
- Steamed broccoli.
- Quinoa.

Day 27:

Breakfast:

- Banana and almond milk smoothie.
- Whole grain toast with a thin spread of cream cheese.

Lunch:

- Turkey and vegetable stir-fry.

- Mixed berry salad.

Dinner:

- Baked chicken with rosemary.
- Roasted sweet potatoes.
- Cauliflower rice.

Day 28:

Breakfast:

- Scrambled eggs with diced tomatoes and spinach.
- Whole grain toast with a thin spread of almond butter.

Lunch:

- Lentil soup with a side of sliced oranges.
- Mixed berry salad.

Dinner:

- Baked chicken breast with herbs.
- Roasted Brussels sprouts.
- Quinoa.

Day 29:

Breakfast:

- Greek yogurt parfait with sliced strawberries and a sprinkle of chopped almonds.

- Whole grain toast with a thin spread of peanut butter.

- Herbal tea.

Lunch:

- Quinoa salad with cherry tomatoes, cucumbers, and feta cheese.

- Sliced melon on the side.

- Green tea.

Dinner:

- Grilled tilapia with a lemon herb marinade.

- Steamed asparagus.

- Brown rice.

Day 30:

Breakfast:

- Smoothie with blueberries, spinach, and low-fat yogurt.

- Whole grain toast with a thin spread of cream cheese.

- Chamomile tea.

Lunch:

- Turkey and avocado wrap with a side of sliced peaches.

- Mixed vegetable sticks.

- Herbal tea.

Dinner:

- Stir-fried tofu with broccoli and snow peas.
- Quinoa.
- Sliced oranges for dessert.

Snack Ideas for a Kidney-Friendly Diet

Enjoying snacks is an important aspect of maintaining a kidney-friendly diet for seniors dealing with kidney stones. Here are some snack ideas broken down for easier understanding:

Fresh Fruit Delight:

- Sliced apples, pears, and berries.
- Optional drizzle of honey for a touch of sweetness.
- Opt for fruits lower in oxalates.

Yogurt Parfait Bliss:

- Low-fat Greek yogurt.
- Moderation is key with chopped nuts (almonds, walnuts).
- Fresh berries for a burst of flavor.
- Sprinkle some ground flaxseeds for added goodness.

Veggie Sticks with Hummus:

- Carrot sticks, cucumber slices, and bell pepper strips.
- Dip into hummus for a tasty and plant-based protein-packed treat.

Cottage Cheese and Pineapple Pleasure:

- Low-fat cottage cheese.

- Enjoy with fresh pineapple chunks.

- Pineapple's bromelain may offer anti-inflammatory benefits.

Protein-Packed Hard-Boiled Eggs:

- A protein-rich option.

- Sprinkle with a pinch of salt and pepper for flavor.

Refreshing Low-Oxalate Smoothie:

- Blend bananas, blueberries, and strawberries.

- Use water or low-fat milk as a base.

- Add ice cubes for a cool and refreshing texture.

Avocado Delight on Rice Cake:

- Brown rice cake.

- Top with sliced avocado.

- Enhance with a dash of lemon juice for taste.

Healthy Popcorn Snack:

- Air-popped popcorn with a modest amount of salt.

- Try a sprinkle of nutritional yeast for added flavor.

Nutty Trail Mix (Remember Portion Control):

- Almonds, pistachios, and dried cranberries.

- Be mindful of portions due to the nut content.

Baked Sweet Potato Fries Treat:

- Sweet potato slices are baked with a touch of olive oil.
- Sprinkle with a pinch of salt and rosemary for a delightful flavor.

Cucumber and Feta Bites:

- Sliced cucumber rounds.
- Top with a small amount of crumbled feta cheese.
- A sprinkle of dill for added taste.

Cherry Tomatoes with Mozzarella Magic:

- Cherry tomatoes paired with fresh mozzarella balls.
- Drizzle with a bit of balsamic glaze for a delightful twist.

Low-Oxalate Berry Sorbet Indulgence:

- Blend mixed berries.
- Freeze the mixture for a homemade sorbet.

Chia Pudding Bliss:

- Mix chia seeds with almond milk.
- Let it sit until it forms a pudding-like consistency.
- Top with sliced kiwi or other low-oxalate fruits.

Tuna on Whole Wheat Crackers:

- Canned tuna (in water) on whole wheat crackers.
- Add a touch of lemon juice for enhanced flavor.

Cooking Tips

Preparation is Key:

- Before you start cooking, make sure to gather all your ingredients.
- Streamline the cooking process by chopping, measuring, and organizing everything in advance.

Knife Skills:

- Efficient and safe chopping begins with mastering basic knife skills.
- Keep your knives sharp for precision and safety.

Mastering Heat:

- Understand your stove or oven settings to control the cooking temperature.
- Medium heat is versatile and works well for many cooking tasks.

Taste as You Go:

- Gradually season your dish and taste frequently to adjust seasoning to your liking.

Balancing Flavors:

- Aim for a well-rounded balance of sweet, salty, sour, and bitter flavors in your dishes.
- Don't be afraid to experiment with different herbs and spices.

Timing Matters:

- Use timers to prevent overcooking and coordinate cooking times for multiple dishes.

Experiment with Herbs and Spices:

- Fresh herbs can add vibrant flavors to your dishes.
- Enhance the aroma of your dishes by toasting spices.

Grains and Pasta:

- Rinse rice before cooking to remove excess starch.
- When boiling pasta, add salt to the water for enhanced flavor.

Protein Perfection:

- Allow meat to rest after cooking to preserve its juiciness.
- Use a meat thermometer for accurate results.

Baking Tips:

- Accurate measurement of ingredients is crucial in baking.
- Ensure consistent results by preheating the oven.

CHAPTER 6

SUPPLEMENTS AND MEDICATIONS

For seniors managing kidney stones, maintaining a diet that's kind to their kidneys involves more than just choosing the right foods. It often means introducing supplements and medications into the mix to bolster overall kidney well-being and keep those stones at bay. Let's delve into the essentials of vitamin and mineral supplements, medications crafted for stone prevention, and the potential dance of interactions and side effects that come with these additions.

Vitamin and Mineral Boosts

a. Calcium Support:

Why? Contrary to what many believe, getting enough calcium is key to keeping kidney stones at bay. However, when it comes to supplements, it's a decision that needs thoughtful consideration.

Tip: Aim to get your calcium from your meals, but if supplements are needed, chat with your healthcare pro for the right dosage.

b. Vitamin D Vitality:

Why? Vitamin D helps your body absorb calcium, and lacking it can pave the way for kidney stones.

Tip: Keep tabs on your vitamin D levels with regular check-ins. If there's a shortfall, your healthcare provider might recommend supplements.

c. Vitamin B6 Buddy:

Why? Vitamin B6 is known to be a stone-stopping force, binding with oxalates in your urine.

Tip: Consider B6 supplements with your healthcare provider's green light as part of your personalized prevention plan.

d. Magnesium Magic:

Why? Magnesium can be a guardian against calcium oxalate crystal formation in your kidneys.

Tip: Opt for magnesium-rich foods when you can, but supplements might be in the cards under your healthcare provider's watchful eye.

Medications for Stone Defense

a. Thiazide Diuretics:

Why? These diuretics, like hydrochlorothiazide, help cut down calcium in your urine, reducing the risk of calcium-based stones.

Tip: When these are in your plan, your healthcare provider will be your guide to ensure they mesh well with your strategy.

b. Allopurinol Ally:

Why? If uric acid stones are your foe, allopurinol might be your ally in lowering uric acid levels in your urine.

Tip: The right dosage and duration? That's a call your healthcare provider will make based on your unique needs.

c. Potassium Citrate Partner:

Why? Potassium citrate can amp up citrate levels in your urine, acting as a stone deterrent.

Tip: Tailored for specific stone types, this one comes with a prescription and a need for careful kidney and electrolyte checks.

Navigating Interactions and Side Effects

a. Calcium and Iron Coordination:

What to Know: Taking calcium and iron supplements together might hamper absorption. Space them out or consider getting iron from your meals.

b. Vitamin D Watch:

What to Know: Too much vitamin D can lead to trouble, from nausea to kidney damage. Keep a close eye on levels to sidestep these issues.

c. Thiazide Diuretic Cautions:

What to Know: These diuretics could bring on dizziness or changes in potassium and blood sugar levels. Regular check-ins with your healthcare provider can keep these in check.

d. Allopurinol Allergies:

What to Know: Allergic reactions, though rare, can range from rashes to severe conditions. If you notice any, seek immediate medical attention.

e. Potassium Citrate and Tummy Tolerance:

What to Know: Some folks might feel a bit queasy with potassium citrate. Adjustments in dosage or form might be needed, under your healthcare provider's guidance.

In wrapping up, weaving supplements and medications into your kidney stone defense plan is no one-size-fits-all venture. It's a personalized journey requiring thoughtful discussions with your healthcare team, regular checks of your health markers, and tweaks based on how your body responds. Before diving into any new regimen, make sure your healthcare team is by your side, steering you toward a plan tailored to your unique needs and ensuring a safe and effective strategy.

CHAPTER 7

ENHANCING KIDNEY HEALTH THROUGH LIFESTYLE CHOICES

When it comes to fostering a lifestyle that supports kidney health, dietary decisions are just a single aspect of the broader picture. This chapter delves into the essential realm of lifestyle adjustments that can profoundly influence the well-being of seniors grappling with kidney stones. We'll delve into the importance of regular physical activity, effective stress management techniques, and the considerable impact of sleep on kidney health.

The Significance of Regular Physical Activity

Regular physical activity isn't only beneficial for cardiovascular health—it plays a pivotal role in bolstering kidney health, particularly for seniors prone to kidney stones. Exercise contributes to overall well-being and can directly and indirectly influence factors affecting kidney stone formation.

Key Aspects of Physical Activity for Kidney Health:

Cardiovascular Exercise:

- Engaging in regular aerobic activities, like walking, jogging, or cycling, enhances blood circulation, promoting optimal kidney function.

- Strive for a minimum of 150 minutes of moderate-intensity exercise each week.

Strength Training:

- Building and preserving muscle mass aids in regulating blood sugar levels and diminishing the risk of metabolic conditions that could contribute to kidney stones.
- Integrate strength training exercises at least twice a week.

Hydration and Exercise:

- Maintaining proper hydration during physical activity is crucial to support kidney function and reduce the risk of stone formation.
- Aim to stay hydrated by drinking water before, during, and after exercise.

Balance and Flexibility:

- Practices such as yoga or tai chi improve balance, flexibility, and overall well-being without imposing excessive strain on the kidneys.

Effective Stress Management Techniques

Chronic stress can profoundly impact overall health, including kidney function. For seniors navigating the challenges of kidney stones, adopting effective stress management techniques is crucial to support not only mental health but also the well-being of the kidneys.

Strategies for Effective Stress Management:

Mindfulness Meditation:

- Mindful meditation techniques can help alleviate stress and promote relaxation, positively impacting kidney health.
- Include short daily meditation sessions for optimal benefits.

Deep Breathing Exercises:

- Deep, diaphragmatic breathing activates the body's relaxation response, mitigating stress.
- Incorporate deep breathing exercises during stressful moments or as part of a daily routine.

Time Management:

- Efficiently managing time and setting realistic goals can prevent feelings of being overwhelmed and stressed.
- Prioritize tasks, delegate when possible, and maintain a balanced schedule.

Social Connections:

- Nurturing strong social connections provides emotional support and serves as a buffer against stress.
- Foster relationships with friends, family, or support groups.

Sleep and Its Impact on Kidney Health

Quality sleep is an often overlooked aspect of overall health, and its significance in kidney health is profound. Poor sleep patterns and inadequate sleep duration can contribute to various health issues, including conditions that may increase the risk of kidney stones.

Optimizing Sleep for Kidney Health:

Consistent Sleep Schedule:

- Maintain a regular sleep-wake cycle to regulate the body's internal clock.
- Aim for 7-9 hours of sleep per night.

Sleep Environment:

- Create a comfortable and dark sleep environment to promote uninterrupted sleep.
- Consider blackout curtains and minimize noise for an optimal sleep setting.

Limiting Stimulants:

- Avoid stimulants like caffeine close to bedtime to ensure a restful sleep.
- Establish a relaxing pre-sleep routine.

Managing Sleep Disorders:

- Address sleep disorders, such as sleep apnea or insomnia, promptly to prevent their impact on kidney health.
- Consult with a healthcare professional for appropriate interventions.

CHAPTER 8

RECIPES FOR KIDNEY STONE-FRIENDLY MEALS

Kidney-friendly breakfast for seniors with kidney stones:

1. Scrambled Egg and Spinach Wrap

Ingredients:

- 2 eggs
- Spinach (limited quantity)
- Whole wheat tortilla

Directions:

- Scramble the eggs in a pan with a little olive oil.
- Add just enough spinach to wilt it.
- Top a whole wheat tortilla with the egg and spinach mixture.

Nutritional Information:

- Calories: 302
- Protein: 12g
- Fiber: 5g

2. Greek Yogurt Parfait

Ingredients:

- Low-fat Greek yogurt

- Sliced apples

- Chopped nuts (almonds, walnuts)

- Ground flaxseeds

Directions:

- In a dish or glass, layer Greek yogurt and sliced apples.

- Sprinkle with ground flaxseeds and chopped nuts.

Nutritional Information:

- Calories: 252

- Protein: 22g

- Fiber: 7g

3. Oatmeal with Berries and Nuts

Ingredients:

- Oatmeal

- Mixed berries

- Chopped nuts (limited quantity)

Directions:

- Cook the oats according to the package directions.

- Finish with a sprinkling of chopped nuts and mixed berries.

Nutritional Information:

- Calories: 204

- Protein: 9g

- Fiber: 7g

4. Cottage Cheese with Peaches

Ingredients:

- Low-fat cottage cheese
- Sliced peaches

Directions:

- Combine low-fat cottage cheese and cut peaches in a mixing bowl.

Nutritional Information:

- Calories: 152
- Protein: 16g
- Fiber: 3g

5. Smoothie with Berries and Almond Milk

Ingredients:

- Berries (blueberries, strawberries)
- Banana
- Almond milk

Directions:

- Until smooth, combine berries, banana, and almond milk.

Nutritional Information:

- Calories: 181
- Protein: 6g
- Fiber: 5g

6. Whole Grain Cereal with Low-Fat Milk

Ingredients:

- Whole grain cereal
- Low-fat milk
- Sliced peaches (optional)

Directions:

- Fill a bowl halfway with whole-grain cereal.
- If desired, top with sliced peaches and low-fat milk.

Nutritional Information:

- Calories: 219
- Protein: 9g
- Fiber: 4g

7. Overnight Oats with Mixed Berries

Ingredients:

- Rolled oats

- Mixed berries
- Low-fat milk

Directions:

- Mix rolled oats with low-fat milk and add mixed berries.
- Refrigerate overnight and enjoy in the morning.

Nutritional Information:

- Calories: 232
- Protein: 8g
- Fiber: 7g

8. Banana and Almond Butter Toast

Ingredients:

- Whole grain toast
- Almond butter
- Sliced banana

Directions:

- Toast the whole-grain bread with almond butter.
- Serve with sliced banana on top.

Nutritional Information:

- Calories: 252
- Protein: 7g
- Fiber: 5g

9. Greek Yogurt with Strawberries

Ingredients:

- Low-fat Greek yogurt
- Sliced strawberries

Directions:

- Combine low-fat Greek yogurt and cut strawberries in a mixing bowl.

Nutritional Information:

- Calories: 181
- Protein: 21g
- Fiber: 4g

10. Smoothie with Spinach and Yogurt

Ingredients:

- Spinach
- Low-fat yogurt
- Banana
- Almond milk

Directions:

- Smoothly combine spinach, low-fat yogurt, banana, and almond milk.

Nutritional Information:

- Calories: 202
- Protein: 9g
- Fiber: 6g

Kidney-friendly lunch for seniors with kidney stones:

1. Grilled Chicken Salad

Ingredients:

- Grilled chicken breast
- Mixed greens
- Cherry tomatoes
- Cucumber
- Olive oil dressing

Directions:

- Grill the chicken breast until it is completely done.
- Mix the mixed greens, cherry tomatoes, and cucumber.
- Drizzle with olive oil dressing and top with grilled chicken.

Nutritional Information:

- Calories: 352
- Protein: 26g
- Fiber: 6g

2. Lentil Soup

Ingredients:

- Lentils
- Mixed vegetables (carrots, celery, onion)
- Low-sodium vegetable broth
- Fresh parsley (optional)

Directions:

- In a saucepan, sauté mixed veggies.
- Combine lentils and low-sodium vegetable broth in a mixing bowl.
- Cook until the lentils are soft. If desired, garnish with fresh parsley.

Nutritional Information:

- Calories: 252
- Protein: 16g
- Fiber: 13g

3. Quinoa Salad with Vegetables

Ingredients:

- Quinoa
- Cherry tomatoes
- Cucumber
- Feta cheese (optional)
- Olive oil dressing

Directions:

- Cook the quinoa according to the package directions.
- Combine quinoa, cherry tomatoes, cucumber, and feta cheese in a mixing bowl.
- Dressing: drizzle with olive oil.

Nutritional Information:

- Calories: 301
- Protein: 11g
- Fiber: 9g

4. Tuna Salad Wrap

Ingredients:

- Canned tuna (in water)
- Whole wheat tortilla
- Mixed greens
- Cherry tomatoes
- Greek yogurt dressing

Directions:

- Combine canned tuna and Greek yogurt dressing in a mixing bowl.
- Fill a whole wheat tortilla with the tuna mixture, mixed greens, and cherry tomatoes.

Nutritional Information:

- Calories: 270
- Protein: 22g
- Fiber: 7g

5. Chickpea Salad

Ingredients:

- Chickpeas (canned, drained)
- Cherry tomatoes
- Feta cheese
- Olive oil dressing

Directions:

- Chickpeas, cherry tomatoes, and feta cheese should all be combined.
- Toss gently with the olive oil dressing.

Nutritional Information:

- Calories: 262
- Protein: 13g
- Fiber: 10g

6. Grilled Salmon with Asparagus

Ingredients:

- Grilled salmon fillet

- Asparagus spears

- Lemon and herbs

Directions:

- Grilled fish with lemon and herbs.

- Steam asparagus till tender.

- Serve the cooked salmon on a bed of asparagus.

Nutritional Information:

- Calories: 322

- Protein: 26g

- Fiber: 5g

7. Vegetable Stir-Fry with Tofu

Ingredients:

- Tofu

- Mixed vegetables (broccoli, bell peppers, snow peas)

- Low-sodium soy sauce

Directions:

- In a skillet, stir-fry tofu and mixed veggies.

- Flavor with low-sodium soy sauce.

Nutritional Information:

- Calories: 284

- Protein: 19g

- Fiber: 8g

8. Quinoa and Black Bean Salad

Ingredients:

- Quinoa

- Black beans (canned, drained)

- Cherry tomatoes

- Lime dressing

Directions:

- Cook the quinoa and set it aside to cool.

- Quinoa, black beans, cherry tomatoes, and lime dressing should be combined.

Nutritional Information:

- Calories: 292

- Protein: 15g

- Fiber: 11g

9. Grilled Shrimp Skewers

Ingredients:

- Shrimp

- Bell peppers

- Zucchini

- Lemon and garlic marinade

Directions:

- Skewers should be threaded with shrimp, bell peppers, and zucchini.
- Grill until the shrimp are cooked through, basting often with the lemon and garlic marinade.

Nutritional Information:

- Calories: 262
- Protein: 22g
- Fiber: 4g

10. Baked Cod with Lemon Herb Marinade

Ingredients:

- Cod fillet
- Lemon and herb marinade
- Steamed broccoli
- Cauliflower rice

Directions:

- Marinate the fish in a lemon-herb mixture.
- Bake until the fish is done. With steamed broccoli and cauliflower rice, serve.

Nutritional Information:

- Calories: 302

- Protein: 24g

- Fiber: 7g

Kidney-friendly dinner for seniors with kidney stones:

1. Baked Chicken Breast with Lemon and Herbs

Ingredients:

- Chicken breast

- Lemon juice

- Fresh herbs (rosemary, thyme)

- Olive oil

- Steamed green beans

- Quinoa

Directions:

- Marinate the chicken breast in lemon juice, fresh herbs, and olive oil.

- Bake until well done. Serve with quinoa and steaming green beans.

Nutritional Information:

- Calories: 322

- Protein: 32g

- Fiber: 6g

2. Vegetable Curry with Chickpeas

Ingredients:

- Mixed vegetables (bell peppers, carrots, peas)
- Chickpeas (canned, drained)
- Curry sauce (low-sodium)
- Cauliflower rice

Directions:

- The curry sauce is used to sauté a variety of vegetables and chickpeas.
- Serve on rice made from cauliflower.

Nutritional Information:

- Calories: 281
- Protein: 13g
- Fiber: 11g

3. Grilled Trout with Lemon and Dill

Ingredients:

- Trout fillet
- Lemon slices
- Fresh dill
- Steamed asparagus

- Brown rice

Directions:

- To grill fish, add slices of lemon and fresh dill to the grill.
- Brown rice and cooked asparagus should be served alongside.

Nutritional Information:

- Calories: 310
- Protein: 26g
- Fiber: 6g

4. Stir-fried vegetables with Tofu

Ingredients:

- Tofu
- Mixed vegetables (broccoli, bell peppers, snow peas)
- Low-sodium soy sauce
- Quinoa

Directions:

- Tofu and a variety of veggies should be stir-fried in a pan.
- Pour in some low-sodium soy sauce. Top with quinoa and serve.

Nutritional Information:

- Calories: 285

- Protein: 19g

- Fiber: 9g

5. Greek Salad with Grilled Salmon

Ingredients:

- Grilled salmon

- Mixed greens

- Cherry tomatoes

- Cucumber

- Feta cheese

- Greek dressing

Directions:

- Grill the salmon, then allow it to cool.

- Prepare a salad consisting of grilled salmon, mixed greens, cherry tomatoes, cucumber, and feta cheese mixture.

- Garnish with Greek dressing and serve.

Nutritional Information:

- Calories: 333

- Protein: 26g

- Fiber: 6g

6. Spinach and Feta-Stuffed Chicken Breast

Ingredients:

- Chicken breast

- Spinach

- Feta cheese

- Lemon juice

- Mixed berry salad

Directions:

- Mix feta cheese and spinach, and then stuff chicken breasts with the mixture.

- Bake until the food is completed. Served with a salad of mixed berries.

Nutritional Information:

- Calories: 311

- Protein: 29g

- Fiber: 7g

7. Quinoa Salad with Tomatoes and Feta

Ingredients:

- Quinoa

- Cherry tomatoes

- Feta cheese

- Olive oil dressing

- Orange slices

Directions:

- Prepare the quinoa and let it cool.

- Quinoa, cherry tomatoes, feta cheese, and olive oil dressing should be combined in a bowl.

- Serve with orange slices as a garnish.

Nutritional Information:

- Calories: 292

- Protein: 11g

- Fiber: 9g

8. Baked Tilapia with Herbs

Ingredients:

- Tilapia fillet

- Lemon and herb marinade

- Roasted Brussels sprouts

- Brown rice

Directions:

- The tilapia should be marinated in a blend of lemon and herbs.

- Bake until the food is completed. The roasted Brussels sprouts and brown rice should be served alongside.

Nutritional Information:

- Calories: 284

- Protein: 23g
- Fiber: 7g

9. Vegetable Stir-Fry with Brown Rice

Ingredients:

- Mixed vegetables (broccoli, carrots, snap peas)
- Low-sodium teriyaki sauce
- Brown rice

Directions:

- Stir-fry a variety of veggies in a teriyaki sauce that is low in salt.
- Serve over a bowl of brown rice.

Nutritional Information:

- Calories: 272
- Protein: 11g
- Fiber: 9g

10. Chickpea and Tomato Salad

Ingredients:

- Chickpeas (canned, drained)
- Cherry tomatoes
- Cucumber
- Olive oil dressing

- Quinoa

Directions:

- The chickpeas, cherry tomatoes, and cucumber should be mixed.
- Olive oil dressing should be drizzled on top. Top with quinoa and serve.

Nutritional Information:

- Calories: 292
- Protein: 14g
- Fiber: 10g

Delicious Desserts without Compromising Kidney Health

1. Berry Parfait

Ingredients:

- Mixed berries (blueberries, strawberries, raspberries)
- Low-fat Greek yogurt
- Chopped nuts (almonds, walnuts)
- Honey (optional)

Directions:

- In a glass, layer a mixture of berries and Greek yogurt with a low-fat content.
- To finish, repeat the layers and sprinkle chopped nuts on top.

- You may drizzle honey on top if you want.

2. Baked Apple with Cinnamon

Ingredients:

- Apple, cored and sliced
- Ground cinnamon
- Chopped nuts (pecans, almonds)
- A touch of honey

Directions:

- The apple slices should be placed in a baking dish.
- Sprinkle with cinnamon and nuts that have been chopped.
- After baking, the apples should be soft. Honey should be drizzled on top before serving.

3. Chia Seed Pudding

Ingredients:

- Chia seeds
- Almond milk (or any low-fat milk)
- Vanilla extract
- Fresh berries for topping

Directions:

- A bowl should be used to combine chia seeds, almond milk, and vanilla essence.

- Put it in the refrigerator until it becomes thick (usually overnight).

- Just before serving, garnish with some fresh berries.

4. Mango Sorbet

Ingredients:

- Ripe mango, peeled and diced

- Lemon or lime juice

- Honey (optional)

Directions:

- To get a smooth consistency, blend chopped mango with lemon or lime juice.

- If more sweetness is required, honey may be used.

- When the mixture is frozen, place it in a shallow pan and stir it periodically until it becomes hard.

5. Watermelon Mint Salad

Ingredients:

- Cubed watermelon

- Fresh mint leaves

- Lime juice

Directions:

- In a bowl, combine watermelon cubes with fresh mint leaves.
- Lemon juice should be drizzled on top before serving.

6. Greek Yogurt with Berries and Almonds

Ingredients:

- Low-fat Greek yogurt
- Mixed berries
- Sliced almonds

Directions:

- Greek yogurt should be poured into a bowl.
- Add a variety of sliced almonds and assorted berries on top.

7. Dark Chocolate-Dipped Strawberries

Ingredients:

- Fresh strawberries
- Dark chocolate (70% cocoa or higher)

Directions:

- Melt dark chocolate in a heatproof bowl.
- Dip each strawberry into the melted chocolate.
- Place on parchment paper to set.

8. Baked Pears with Cinnamon

Ingredients:

- Ripe pears, halved and cored
- Ground cinnamon
- Chopped walnuts
- A touch of honey

Directions:

- A baking dish should be filled with pear halves.
- The cinnamon and chopped walnuts should be sprinkled on top.
- Roast the pears until they are soft. Honey should be drizzled on top before serving.

9. Frozen Banana Bites

Ingredients:

- Bananas, sliced
- Natural peanut butter
- Unsweetened shredded coconut

Directions:

- The banana slices should be spread with peanut butter.
- Stack them on top of one another and then roll them in shredded coconut.
- Put in the freezer until solid.

10. Lemon Sorbet

Ingredients:

- Freshly squeezed lemon juice
- Water
- Sweetener (optional)

Directions:

- Lemon juice should be combined with water and, if necessary, sugar.
- When the mixture is frozen, place it in a shallow pan and stir it periodically until it becomes hard.

The Role of Dietitians in Kidney Stone Management

In the intricate landscape of kidney stone management, dietitians emerge as invaluable partners, offering personalized guidance to navigate the dietary intricacies that contribute to kidney stone formation. This chapter delves into the pivotal role of dietitians in empowering individuals with tailored nutritional strategies, fostering a holistic approach to kidney stone prevention and management.

Assessment and Personalized Nutrition Plans:

- Understanding the Individual: Dietitians conduct thorough assessments, considering factors like age, lifestyle, medical history, and stone composition.

- Tailored Nutrition Plans: Leveraging their expertise, dietitians craft customized nutrition plans, emphasizing the restriction or inclusion of specific nutrients based on individual requirements.

Dietary Modifications for Stone Prevention:

- Fluid Intake Guidance: Dietitians provide precise recommendations on fluid intake to ensure adequate hydration, a cornerstone in preventing stone formation.
- Calcium Management: Dispelling myths, dietitians guide individuals on optimizing calcium intake through dietary sources while minimizing supplements, striking a delicate balance for stone prevention.

Oxalate and Sodium Management:

- Oxalate-Aware Diets: With a nuanced understanding of oxalate-rich foods, dietitians help structure diets that manage oxalate levels effectively.
- Sodium Restriction: Recognizing the role of sodium in stone formation, dietitians educate on sodium awareness, offering practical strategies for sodium restriction.

Protein Moderation and Acid-Base Balance:

- Protein-Related Considerations: Dietitians address the impact of excessive animal protein on stone risk, emphasizing moderation and diversification.

- Acid-Base Balance: With an understanding of acid-base equilibrium, dietitians guide individuals in balancing acid-forming and alkaline-forming foods for optimal kidney health.

Monitoring and Adjustment:

- Regular Dietary Monitoring: Dietitians advocate for ongoing dietary monitoring, ensuring that nutritional plans evolve in tandem with individual responses and changing health conditions.
- Adjustment Strategies: When needed, dietitians adeptly modify nutrition plans, accommodating shifting dietary needs or addressing new health considerations.

Collaboration with Healthcare Teams:

- Multidisciplinary Approach: Dietitians seamlessly collaborate with urologists, nephrologists, and other healthcare professionals, contributing their expertise to a multidisciplinary approach.
- Educational Support: Beyond individual consultations, dietitians engage in educational initiatives, empowering individuals and healthcare providers with the latest nutritional insights.

Empowering Lifestyle Changes:

- Beyond Diet: Recognizing the interconnectedness of health, dietitians champion comprehensive lifestyle changes, including physical activity, stress management, and adequate sleep, fostering a holistic approach to kidney stone management.

Dealing with Challenges in Adhering to the Diet Plan

Starting a kidney stone diet plan might be life-changing, but it's not without difficulties. In this chapter, we address frequent challenges that people may encounter and provide doable solutions to ensure long-term adherence to your customized kidney stone diet.

Social Contexts and Eating Outside:

- **The Secret is to Prepare:** Prepare ahead of time for social gatherings. Inform the restaurant staff or hosts about any dietary restrictions.
- **Wise Decisions:** Make intelligent food selections by choosing kidney stone-friendly items. Pick salads, grilled meats, and foods with little to no additional salt.

Temptations and Cravings:

- **Find healthy alternatives** to your favorite snacks that won't cause kidney stones. For instance, choose a fruit sorbet over ice cream.

- **Moderation:** Give yourself little indulgences from time to time. The secret is to balance pleasures with strict dietary compliance.

Limited Choices or Preferences for Food:

- **Diversify Your Options:** To keep your meals interesting and fulfilling, try a range of foods that are suitable for kidney stones.
- **Recipe Adjustment:** Make sure you enjoy your favorite foods without jeopardizing the health of your kidneys by adjusting recipes to suit your dietary requirements.

Convenience foods and time constraints:

- **Meal Prep:** Set aside time to prepare meals, with an emphasis on kidney stone-friendly dishes. For hectic days, prepare and freeze meals.
- **Options for Healthful Snacks:** Store easily accessible, low-fat snacks nearby to avoid giving in to the lure of less healthy options.

Stress and Emotional Consumption:

- **Eating With Awareness:** Learn to identify genuine hunger from emotional stimulants by engaging in mindful eating. Before grabbing for food, take a moment to evaluate your emotions.

- **Techniques for Stress Management:** Take up stress-relieving exercises like meditation, deep breathing, or a quick stroll to address emotional eating habits.

Traveling Difficulties:

- **Think Before You Pack:** When traveling, pack meals and snacks that won't cause kidney stones. Before traveling, check out the food selections in your location.
- **Maintain Hydration:** Keep yourself well-hydrated while traveling, since this is a critical component in preventing kidney stones.

Lack of Advancement or Plateau:

- **Reevaluate and Adjust:** Discuss your food plan with your healthcare team or dietician if you are not improving. Adaptations can be required in light of your changing health requirements.
- **Honor Non-Scale Achievements:** Acknowledge benefits that go beyond measurements, including more energy or improved general well-being.

Absence of Assistance:

- **Communication:** Explain to your loved ones the significance of your kidney stone diet plan by sharing your dietary objectives with them.

- **Find Supportive Communities:** To exchange experiences and guidance, and make connections with others going through comparable struggles online or in local support groups.

CHAPTER 9

CONCLUSION

As we conclude this illuminating trip through the "Kidney Stone Diet for Seniors," it's critical to consider the most important lessons learned and reaffirm our dedication to living a kidney-friendly lifestyle. This chapter urges a firm commitment to maintaining kidney health into old age by providing a thorough summary of the most important lessons learned throughout the book.

Summary of the Main Points

Knowing About Kidney Stones:

- **Factors of Formation:** Review the elements that lead to kidney stone development, such as food, underlying medical disorders, and dehydration.

- **Stone Types:** List the common kinds of kidney stones and stress how important it is to determine which kind to avoid to develop specialized preventative measures.

- **Dietary Guidelines for the Kidney Stone Diet:** To lower the chance of a stone recurrence, review the dietary recommendations and pay particular attention to low-oxalate, low-sodium, and appropriate fluid consumption.

Emphasize the significance of attaining a balanced consumption of foods high in oxalate and calcium.

Organizing Meals:

- **Balanced Meals:** Use a range of foods that are favorable to kidney stones to reinforce the idea of creating balanced meals.
- **Emphasize the need for portion management**, particularly for meals that are rich in salt or oxalates.

Nutrition Information Labels:

- **Label Reading:** Tell elders to practice reading nutrition labels so they can spot additives and hidden salt sources.

Hydration:

- **Water Consumption:** Stress the importance of being well-hydrated as the first line of defense against kidney stones.
- **Flexible Decisions:** Promote drinking water instead of caffeinated or sugar-filled drinks.
- **Vitamin D and Calcium Supplements and Drugs:** Describe the need to preserve ideal vitamin D levels and the balanced approach to calcium use.

Emphasize the role that drugs like potassium citrate and thiazide diuretics play in preventing stones.

Changes in Lifestyle:

- **Engaging in Exercise:** Emphasize the advantages of regular exercise for general health and renal health.
- **Stress Management:** Stress-reduction tactics like deep breathing and mindfulness should be emphasized.
- **Good Sleep:** Remind elderly people of the significant influence good sleep has on renal health.

Handling Difficulties:

- **Social Situations:** Provide advice on how to follow the kidney stone diet while attending social gatherings and eating out.
- **Cravings and Temptations:** Promote moderation in the odd indulgence without sacrificing nutritional objectives.
- **Time Restraints and Travel:** Offer helpful advice for sticking to the diet while on the go and with hectic schedules.

Adopting a Kidney-Friendly Way of Life

- **Individual Promise:** Evaluate Your Progress: Motivate elders to evaluate their experiences and recognize the strides they have made in following the kidney stone diet.
- **Establishing Achievable Objectives:** Stress the need to establish attainable goals to maintain success.

- **Creating a Network of Support:** Friends and Family: Emphasize how important a supportive atmosphere is to sustaining a lifestyle that is good for the kidneys.
- **Healthcare Team:** Remind elders to continue interacting with their healthcare team and to ask for advice and modifications as necessary.

Long-Term View:

- **Dedicated Lifetime:** Reiterate the notion that maintaining kidney health requires a lifetime of careful consideration of one's food and lifestyle choices.
- **Advocate for regular health examinations** to track kidney function and evaluate the success of the preventative strategy.

Honoring Achievement:

- **Non-Scale Victories:** Honor accomplishments that go beyond the scale, such as more vitality, a happier disposition, and better general health.
- **Community Involvement:** Promote involvement in forums or groups where people discuss their achievements and difficulties in maintaining kidney health.

- **Scientific Progress:** Draw attention to the ongoing developments in kidney stone research, which provide hope for better methods of care and prevention.
- **Adapting to Change:** Tell elders to keep up with any changes to dietary recommendations so they may modify their programs appropriately.

As we wrap off this thorough guide, we honor seniors' commitment to achieving the best possible renal health. Through the adoption of the main insights and dedication to a kidney-friendly way of living, every person can ensure a better, more satisfying life throughout their older years. Seniors may take proactive measures to protect their health, as seen by their tenacity and dedication in implementing and adhering to the kidney stone diet. I hope that this last chapter will encourage a fresh commitment to renal health and a bright and happy future for all.

www.ingramcontent.com/pod-product-compliance
Lightning Source LLC
Chambersburg PA
CBHW060945260726
48661CB00005B/1762